4 Pitfalls & Traps That Prevent Lasting Health:

How to feel confident about your health, maintain your quality of life and ensure that you NEVER again feel the way you did when you first walked into our clinic.

Study Version

ISBN: 9781073100323

Contact: Norman Lowrey, Alternative Health Atlanta
1640 Powers Ferry Rd., Building 14 Suite 100, Marietta, GA 30067
770-937-9200
Email: Norman@AlternativeHealthAtlanta.com
Website: www.AlternativeHealthAtlanta.com

Disclaimer: The information in this book is designed to provide helpful information on the subjects discussed. This book is not meant to be used, nor should it be used, to diagnose or treat any medical condition. For diagnosis or treatment of any medical problem, consult your own physician. The publisher and author are not responsible for any specific health needs or conditions that may require medical supervision and are not liable for any damages or negative consequences from any treatment, action, application, or preparation, to any person reading or following the information in this book. References are provided for informational purposes only and do not constitute endorsement of any websites or other sources. Readers should be aware that the websites listed in this book may change.

Attention: Quantity discounts and customized versions of this book are available for bulk purchases. For permission requests or quantity discounts, please email Norman Lowrey at Norman@AlternativeHealthAtlanta.com

Printed in the United States of America

Contents

4 Pitfalls & Traps That Prevent Lasting Health

Preface

Health care professionals, researchers, government health agencies, health statisticians, and health writers all agree that most chronic health problems could be resolved or improved if people would live a healthy lifestyle.

Well, as you know, most people won't!

But I've found that there is a special group, a niche, that will sometimes buck the trend, live a healthy lifestyle, and stay healthy for the rest of their lives. The good news? If you're holding this book, then you belong to this small, esoteric niche!

You qualify because:

1. You have found a natural solution to chronic health problems that's outside of conventional drug treatment.
2. By doing an Evectics^{SM} program, you took on the personal responsibility of getting your own health back and helping your body to heal, instead of looking for a medical "fix."
3. It worked! You have proven that your body can heal with specific, targeted assistance and improved diet and lifestyle— when conventional treatment had failed.

I've observed that this group (you!) with these common experiences also have the motivation of never, ever wanting to return to the condition that prompted them to come to us in the first place.

> **But despite this motivation, most of this group—your group—will end up in health trouble all over again.**
>
> *This short book is dedicated to preventing this from occurring in your specific case.*

It's entirely possible that this book could have a huge impact on the remainder of your life.

Well, what have you got to lose? It will take you all of 30 minutes to read it!

I wish you excellent health for the rest of your life.

Norman Lowrey

What is Evectics℠?

Evectics℠ is a *"holistic whole-health solution."* The goal of Evectics℠ is *to help patients with chronic health problems so that their body is no longer a problem in their life, for the rest of their life.*

Evectics℠ includes solutions for every phase of your recovery:

1. Help the body to reverse severe chronic conditions and begin to improve, instead of worsening
2. Help the body to stabilize itself and begin to heal
3. Assist the body to de-stress and heal the causes that created the chronic conditions
4. Monitor and maintain improving health in patients for the rest of their lives, despite any permanent damage from previous chronic conditions

For more information on Evectics℠, visit our website at https://alternativehealthatlanta.com/

Or read Dr. Billiot's book:

How to Avoid the Medical Tiger Trap and Get Your Life Back

(Available from the clinic or from Amazon)

There's a TOP to the CHART!
Don't fall off

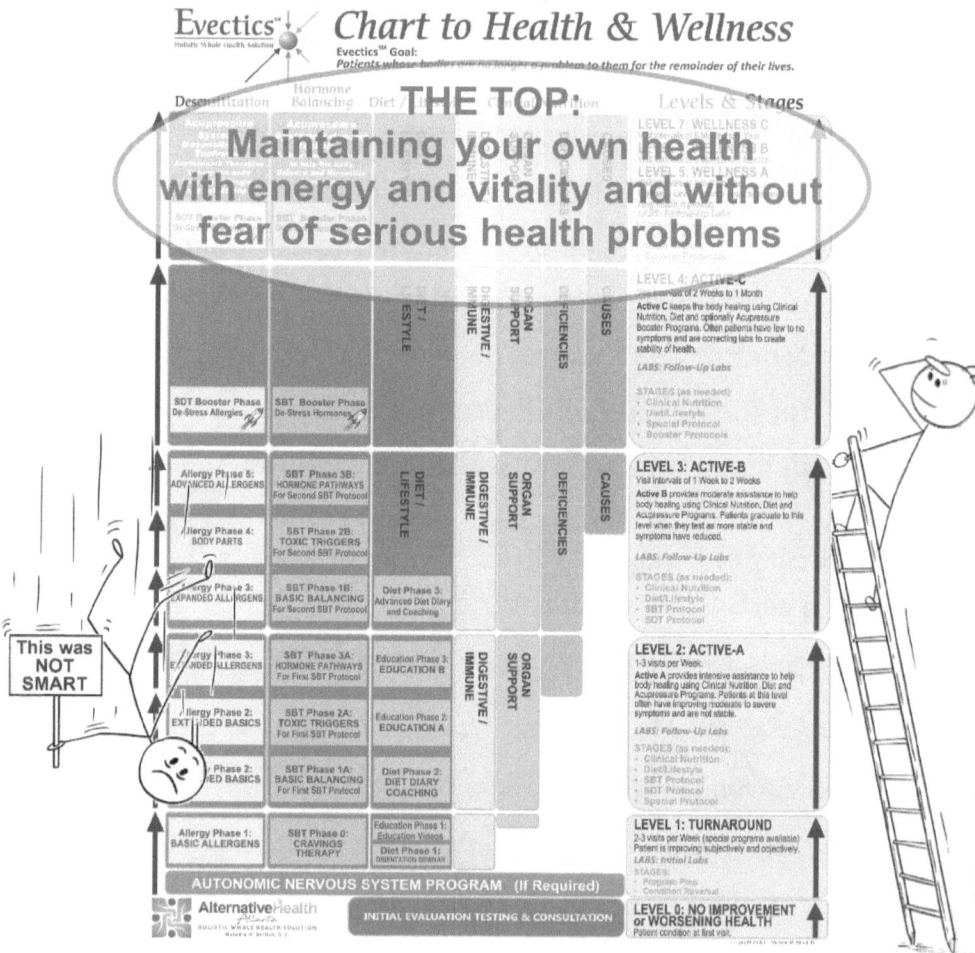

The Evectics[SM] Chart to Health and Wellness is an innovation in health care. Based on research and observation of how bodies heal, the chart shows how health is recovered level by level.

Congratulations!

You've started an Evectics℠ program, done the hard work, and have successfully changed the direction of your health—and quite possibly your life. You have, through your own efforts and actions, reversed your worsening health toward an improving condition.

This by itself would be considered a near miracle by many in the medical field. Their expectations for chronic patients such as yourself are that you will continue to take drugs to control and manage symptoms . . . for the rest of your life. They also fully expect that your health will continue to decline, and that you will need to be treated with additional drugs and possibly surgeries from now on.

But . . .

No matter how miraculous some MD might find your recovery, you may not see it quite that way. My experience with patients is that they are happy—sometimes *very* happy—that they feel better. But "miracle?" Well, maybe not. You probably aren't waking up daily like Scrooge on Christmas morning, leaping and dancing about, celebrating your wonderful new health (my apologies if this does describe you!).

4 Pitfalls & Traps That Prevent Lasting Health

In my experience, most patients adapt pretty quickly to their new health. If anything, their attention goes to those issues that haven't completely improved while they mostly forget about or take for granted the symptoms that got better.

This can be true even when there have been dramatic improvements.

It's an interesting observation I've made: most people who are mid-process in recovering from a long-term health problem—one that they may at one time have considered to be ruining their life—don't necessarily stay interested in continuing the process once their symptoms improve enough to not be an overwhelming concern.

> **I've seen that people who stick with a health improvement program long enough to become stably healthy are not at all common.**

Study Question Box 1

1. What would you consider is your biggest health improvement on your Evectics^{SM} program so far?

2. Are you less concerned about this problem than when you first started with us?

3. Write out your own goal for your health. Include short- and long-term goals, with long-term being the rest of your life.

    SHORT TERM:

    LONG TERM:

I'll make you a deal.

Read the rest of what I have to say here about how to avoid going back to the situation that brought you to us in the first place. If you do this, I promise to shoot completely straight with you. I've learned some useful information by watching patients succeed and fail for 25 years, and I'll give you the straight scoop, no moral lessons, no embellishment. I also won't preach. It's YOUR life, YOUR body, and YOUR health.

First, let's establish the goal. How about this for a goal: to fully recover your health so you have a high quality of life, don't worry about your health anymore, and NEVER again feel the way you did when you first walked into our clinic?

Are you interested in avoiding the traps and pitfalls that could prevent you from achieving this?

Yes? OK, here we go.

The 4 Pitfalls and Traps that Prevent Stable, Long-Term Health:

4 Pitfalls & Traps That Prevent Lasting Health

Pitfall and Trap #1: "Negative Gain" and Ancient Body Design

Negative Gain: *Getting rid of something that you never wanted in the first place.*

You may at some time in your life have had some serious pain from an injury, burn, headache, or hangover. This would have been the "You can have my kingdom if I can get rid of this pain" kind of pain. Your whole world was wrapped up in enduring it. Then, the next morning it was mostly or completely gone. I'll bet that within a few hours you had almost forgotten about it. Surely, a week later you weren't walking around constantly thankful that you didn't have the pain anymore. It's *negative gain*: you got rid of something that you never wanted to have.

> With *negative gain*, you may be highly motivated to solve your problem . . . right up to the point that it gets somewhat better. Then you may forget about it and refocus on some other problem that now seems more important.

The thing to know about negative gain is that a person will mostly or completely *forget* the problem ever happened, which can lead to relapses in the behaviors that caused the problem originally. This can result in the problem coming back. This is one of the reasons we have you do surveys every visit to track changes in your symptoms. It's not at all uncommon to ask a patient about a change in a symptom and hear, "It hasn't changed very much, it was never very bad." I'm looking at their symptom survey, where they marked a "10" (worst possible) at their first visit. How was this "never very bad?" Often, I'll have to go back to their original history form and read them what they wrote to get them to recall it! It might say something like, "I can't get to sleep or stay asleep, I wake in the morning exhausted. I am afraid I will lose my job because I'm so tired all day." To see the genuine surprise this causes is to realize the power of negative gain to erase memory.

Theft of Your Regained Sense of Health and Optimism

As your body regains its ability to heal, it recovers and comes out of a state of deterioration. It may not seem like it to you, but when you are failing to heal and getting worse, your body is actually *dying* by degrees. This reduces not only physical energy but affects mental attitude and viewpoint as well. Life isn't as interesting, and it can be an effort to live it.

4 Pitfalls & Traps That Prevent Lasting Health

The clinic staff is always remarking on this: new patients a month or so into their programs start to look healthier, brighter, and happier. They often become friendlier and more communicative, their color changes, and they may even start dressing better!

Negative gain claims this new well-being as its first victim. Often this isn't a symptom you had voiced as a problem, and it's horribly easy to essentially "get your life back" and then not even know it happened!

Negative gain by itself can cause you problems with maintaining your health, but when you combine it with how your body handles symptoms and stress, *you have a recipe for disaster.*

You have the same body as a caveman. OK, maybe a cavewoman. Regardless, this is true. Bodies haven't been updated or redesigned for roughly 200,000 years. We're still on version 1.0. Back in the early days, there were no doctors, so anything that went wrong with health just had to get better on its own. The body healed itself or died. No other options were available. Back then, having a symptom could be very dangerous. If Joe Caveman suffered from chronic migraines, he'd be distracted by his pain and quickly gobbled up by something hungry or bashed in by a rival caveman (woman).

> **To improve survival, Mother Nature designed bodies to hide symptoms for as long as possible.**

If stress becomes too overwhelming, the body is forced to show a symptom. However, once the body has a symptom, *any improvement that reduces the stress will allow the body to hide the symptom as a first action,* even before it attempts to heal the cause of the problem. Hiding the symptom improves the chances of survival, and there is no point in trying to heal something if you aren't going to survive.

(IMPORTANT FACT: Bodies will hide a symptom as soon as any stress reduction makes this possible. Therefore, a symptom improving does NOT mean that the cause of the symptom has healed, though it does show there is less stress in the area.)

That was all fine back then, but this is still how your body behaves 2,000 centuries later!

If you've had a health problem for several years, have started a program with us within the last six months or so, and now feel much better, *your body is hiding the symptoms and has just started the healing process!* Proof of this will usually show in your Tissue Mineral Analysis lab. I'm not telling you that you aren't hugely improved. The fact that your body is successfully able to compensate for (hide) many of your past symptoms is proof of this.

I understand that you may feel that you are truly healed from your problems. Hang in there and hear me out. Your future health may depend on this.

A caveman body with negative gain symptom improvement is a setup for the relapse of your health problems. Negative gain has erased the memory of how your health used to mess up your life, but the improvement you are experiencing will be temporary unless you continue to work hard to keep your body healing. But why should you? Now you're in danger of joining the group of our patients who stop supporting their health, believing incorrectly that they won't relapse into problems again ("What problems? I feel fine").

Study Question Box 2

1. Give an example from your life of negative gain (a problem that went away and you forgot it ever happened, or it seems like a much smaller problem than when you had it).

2. Did you have a symptom when you first started your program that you might be in the process of forgetting about? If so, what is it?

3. Based on the information that your body is still a "caveman," when a symptom you had previously improves or goes away, does this mean:

   ❑ That area of your body has completely healed.
   ❑ Your body is healing the area.
   ❑ Your body is hiding the symptom and may just be starting to heal the area.

Actual Experience: *What Happens When You Leave Your Treatment Program Incomplete*

Many patients stop their health improvement programs long before they have healed enough to be stable, or they slip back into old stressful lifestyles. In either case, this added stress will overcome any benefits from all the work they did previously or any reduced treatment program they may have continued.

This can result in several different outcomes. Here's what often happens:

- **The original symptoms return** several years later. We always have patients who return for care when their health "falls apart" a few years after stopping their programs. If the symptoms return in a short time, this may cause the patient to realize they really weren't "done" with their program, but this can also create buyer's remorse. The person may decide that our program didn't work. After all, the problem came back!

- **The patient feels much better and quits** our program. Who in their right mind would go to a doctor if they felt well? (Especially if there's no insurance coverage.) Over time, symptoms gradually start to show up. The patient looks around, and everyone they see has similar symptoms. They think, "Hey, this must be normal—after all, I'm in my 40s!" The patient does the "normal" thing and gets on several drugs. Ten years later, this person has "normal" (awful) health* and there is *no remaining benefit from the time, education, effort, and finance they invested in their Evectics*^{SM} *program.*

AARP did an online survey in 2016 of 1,800 adults over the age of 50. Among survey respondents, **75 percent took a prescription medication on a regular basis, with an even higher percentage for those ages 65 and older. Of these, over 80 percent took at least two prescription drugs and over 50 percent take four or more.*

- **Completely different symptoms begin** anywhere from months to years after stopping a program. This is a trap, because the person thinks that with *different* symptoms, there must be a completely different problem that has nothing to do with their previous treatment program with us. They will search for a solution, usually starting with medicine (it's paid for by insurance). Sometimes, they won't think that we can help with these new and different symptoms and never call. Often, they think that since the problem "just started" it can be quickly and inexpensively (with insurance) "fixed" with a drug. They came to us in the first place because of a long-term problem that medicine failed to help, and medicine hasn't failed yet with this new problem. In most cases the symptoms are different, but the cause is the same one that brought them to us originally, and medical treatment will just stress their body even more. Sadly, this may be the beginning of the end of the lifelong good health they had begun to create.

> **"Different Symptoms" Example** (just had two of these, by the way): Patient Jane Smith "fully recovers" her health on our program ("fully recovered" = "her symptoms are gone"). She quits her treatment program since she's "done." A few years later, she develops dangerous high blood pressure, gets put on three drugs, then starts to exhibit other symptoms (diabetes), which are treated medically as well. Jane remembers that we helped her before and comes back to us. Upon testing, we find that Jane has the same weaknesses and stresses left over from her original incomplete program. With lifestyle changes, supplements, and acupressure, Jane's

doctor takes her off her meds, and she is back into a healing state within a few months. *Compare this outcome to where she was headed medically with lifelong drug therapy: kidney failure, nerve damage and loss of extremities, stroke, heart disease, etc.*

Priorities

Patients who drop out of treatment and relapse in one way or another usually make their error based on priorities.

Your health can stop being a priority in your life when your symptoms improve enough to where you can live with them. With other things in your life now becoming your main priority, you may stop the actions you were doing to recover your health.

This is a problem, because once your body has suffered from a significant chronic health condition of any kind, you will need to adjust your life permanently in order to supply the extra support required to maintain your health.

> **In order to avoid having your health problem be your main priority in your life, you will have to make taking care of your health a main priority in your life.**

Study Question Box 3

1. Your best friend just went through a health scare episode with pain, weakness, and dizziness. The doctor says nothing shows up, the problem got better, and your friend is telling you how happy he is that this is all behind him now. What would be some advice you might give to your friend?

2. If you dropped out of care with us before you were stable and then developed symptoms a year later that were different from the symptoms you had while a patient with us, what could this mean?

3. If you continued to do a treatment program with us even though most of your symptoms had improved or gone away, would it mean:
    - ❏ You were foolish and being taken advantage of.
    - ❏ Your body can hide your symptoms but has not completed healing the underlying causes. Continuing a program allows your body to finish the job.
    - ❏ You were well, but kept your treatment going just to be sure nothing else happened to damage your health.

Pitfall and Trap #2: A Definition of Insanity

Einstein is credited with the quote, "Insanity is doing the same thing over and over again and expecting a different result." A slight variation of this would be, "Insanity is acting the same as everyone else and expecting to have a different outcome than theirs."

Dr. Billiot's book *Get Your Life Back* makes a very strong case about how common chronic disease is in our society. CDC statistics show about half the population is suffering from a serious chronic condition. Don't take their word for it. Go for a walk down a crowded street or in a crowded store or restaurant and *look*:

- How many people are overweight? (maybe half or more?)

- How many of those overweight people do you think probably have high blood pressure or diabetes?

- Look at some faces. How many appear happy and healthy? Stressed out? Drugged? Obviously ill with something?

- How many people are not walking in an energetic, coordinated, and pain-free way?

4 Pitfalls & Traps That Prevent Lasting Health

If you did this assignment, you will understand my point very well, indeed. Now think through the list of people you know well. How many of them have chronic illness and are on drugs long term?

Question: If you live the way these people do, eat the way they do, do healthcare the way they do, are you imagining that you won't be like them?

I understand that having a healthy lifestyle is inconvenient. No fast food. Little sugar. No junk food. Gee . . . can't we just have a little fun here? What's the big deal? (This attitude is what your uninitiated friends and family are almost surely going to think and say, and they can be VERY convincing, especially when bringing you potato chips and beer). But what if this was the only way to avoid long-term health problems? *What if it was?*

Study Question Box 4

1. "Most people in their 50s and 60s will need to be on at least one or two long-term drugs just because of their age." Is this statement true?
   - ❏ Yes, it's true
   - ❏ Not true but based on the statistics, a person would need to be very proactive to avoid this.

2. How many people do you know that have chronic health conditions? (Diabetes, high blood pressure, heart disease, arthritis, depression, COPD, overweight, fatigue) _____

3. "More than half the population suffers from chronic illness and over 30% of everyone you know will die from heart disease." *Severe health problems will NOT happen in your future because:* (Write why not)

Pitfall and Trap #3: "I want someone to fix me"

If you are caught in this trap, you've succumbed to the idea that there is a "fix" for your problem, and that you just need to find it!

> **The truth is, there is no "fix" to a chronic health condition, if "fix" is defined as "quick and someone else does if for me."**

The belief that there is a "fix" to a long-term health problem is partly rooted in drug company marketing. All drug ads push the line, "If you have symptoms, you are sick and need treatment (drugs). If your symptoms lessen or go away with the drug, now you are healthy (even if you have to continue to take the drug)." Every drug ad shows happy people recovered from their problems because they are taking a drug. This is the thinking that allows a person to take a drug for high blood pressure every day for the rest of his life and believe that he doesn't have a health problem. This same person might believe that his high blood pressure went away as soon as he started the drug, and that now it's *fixed!* The truth is that the drug only suppresses the symptom, leaving the underlying condition to worsen, and stresses the body with a toxic drug.

4 Pitfalls & Traps That Prevent Lasting Health

Chronic health conditions evolve over many years. You may have had health problems for a decade or more before you had symptoms. Your body is very, very good at compensating, working around problems, and hiding symptoms. By the time it runs out of options and can't hide the stresses from you any longer, there is a lot of damage to repair, which will usually take it many years to accomplish. **There's no "quick fix" available because the problem took years to develop and simply can't be fixed quickly**.

There is only healing, which takes time and discipline from you. The longer you believe in the "fix fiction," the longer it will take you to get started on the process of healing (if you ever do). Meanwhile, your condition will likely continue to worsen.

Chronic health conditions take a long time to develop and a long time to heal. A rule of thumb on this would be at least three months of healing for every year you have been aware of your problem.

Getting "fixed" medically is very alluring. The whole concept is fabulous marketing: "No effort on your part! Just take this drug! Insurance will pay!"

The Most Common "Fix-Me Trap" Mistake

"Try medicine first, do the difficult 'healthy lifestyle' thing only if it doesn't work."

In my experience, this one is so common it's almost a given. A past patient comes in and says, "Well, a year after I stopped coming to you (because I felt so great), I started having this tingling in my fingers and toes. It got pretty bad, so I had it checked out by my doctor and, wow, I was pre-diabetic! But he said not to worry, I wasn't a diabetic yet, and if I took this drug it might prevent that."

Me: "Did the drug help with your tingling?"

Patient: "Well, no. That's one reason I came back to you. He couldn't find any reason for the tingling."

Don't misunderstand me, there are a lot of good reasons to get checked out by a competent medical doctor if you develop a symptom. You want to rule out any immediate medical danger that a doctor could and should handle. **But you might want to find out if there is a solution that will help your body to heal from whatever your doctor is diagnosing, rather than agreeing to a lifetime of drugs and worsening health.** *Remember, your medical doctor most often won't know there's any other solution* *(much less one that would work) and will often believe that his way is the only way.*

Why is this? Why can't there be a "fix?"

"Chronic health conditions take a long time to develop and a long time to heal." –Dr. Billiot.

Once again, why this is true?

> **Because drugs do not handle the *causes* of chronic health problems.**

It all goes back to the caveman concept. Your body is designed to keep itself operational with no help from outside. When your body gets stressed (from a bacteria or virus, an allergy, toxins, etc.) it will try to resolve that stress. If it fails to resolve the stress completely, it will adapt as much as possible to continue to operate despite the stress.

Stress that your body is forced to adapt to because it can't heal completely is called a *cause*. Causes (usually several) create chronic health problems. **A chronic health problem is what your body is forced to do to adapt**

and keep living despite the stress of one or more causes.

So, if you want your chronic health problem to end, you will have to help your body fully resolve any causes it is living with.

Causes: *virus, bacteria, fungus, chemical toxins, heavy metal toxins, allergies, radiation, and a few more rare ones.*

Helping your body recover from causes isn't short term, quick 'n' easy, or "fixable." But it IS possible!

By the way: These causes are weak points in your body. When you add stress to your lifestyle, you make these causes worse and slow the healing process.

Stress sources: Bad diet habits (sugar, junk food, refined carbohydrates, alcohol), associating with toxic personalities, not sleeping enough, not helping your body heal by taking recommended supplements, or missing appointments with us.

Study Question Box 5

1. Think of an experience you've had in your life where you wanted a "fix" for a situation you found yourself in. Recall how you realized there was no "fix" and instead took responsibility and handled the situation yourself with a good result. You can share if you like!

2. Most people will "try medicine first" for a health problem. Getting checked out medically is a great idea, but there are two types of recommendations you may receive (see below). Which of these would you want to get checked by an Evectics^{SM} doctor before submitting to medical treatment?
   - ❑ "Your problem is XXX-itis. With this short drug treatment, you'll be right as rain."
   - ❑ "Your problem is YYY-itis. You will need to take this drug for the rest of your life / you will need this surgery.

Pitfall and Trap #4: The Value-of-Health Equation

Value-of-Health Equation: *"Relief of today's symptom is not worth the money and time required for stable, long-term health."*

In this trap, the person fails to accurately predict the future and makes decisions based only on how they feel right now.

This is the same reason it's hard for people to save money for the future. They have enough right now and don't really want to look too closely at what their future needs could be or take the sometimes-painful steps to make sure they're prepared.

I see this trap in action frequently. Me: "So, here is the program that the doctor is recommending for you to stabilize your health and continue healing."

Patient: "Wow, that's expensive and time-consuming. I don't know if I can do that."

Me: "Don't worry, I have several approaches to getting you to a stable condition. You can do it fast or slow, depending on the finances and time you have available."

Patient: "I'll have to think about it." (This actually means, "I have compared the symptoms I still have with the time and money you are saying I'll have to spend, and the value-of-health equation doesn't add up. I am OK living with my current condition if I can avoid spending the time and money to make it better.")

Patients who are improved but still have serious symptoms will continue their health improvement programs. Patients who have improved most of their important symptoms will usually not. Their decision is based on comparing their current symptoms with the time and money needed to continue their program. **Future health problems aren't considered because the patient assumes that if the symptom is gone, the problem causing it has also gone.** When a patient ends a treatment program before his health is stable, it usually leads to a reversal and worsening of the person's health condition.

> **Their efforts and finances spent so far will be sacrificed over the next years as they return to chronic health problems.**

I hate to put it that way; it seems so dire. Yet, after 25 years of watching patients, I have no doubt that this is EXACTLY what occurs.

Value-of-Health Equation and Labs

Here's what most of us know about lab tests:

- They cost too much.
- They are unpleasant to do.
- They are confusing to understand.
- Sometimes they contain bad news.

So, what's not to like?

Actually, there's quite a lot to like.

What's the purpose of a lab test?

A lab objectively measures the result of something your body does. It measures the *result* of a body function. The lab doesn't show what is there, it shows what your body is *doing*. We often call the labs we use "functional labs" for this reason.

A medical doctor uses labs to put you on a drug.

When your medical doctor looks at your labs, he's got no choice but to guess what is causing the lab value. It is likely he'll just put you on an appropriate drug to correct the lab. This is because medical doctors mainly treat symptoms. An out-of-range lab is a symptom, and a drug is designed to control or suppress a symptom.

We use labs to guide nervous system testing in order to find out what your body most wants help with.

When we look at your labs, it shows us an area that is or is not functioning properly. This is information that we use to test with. Because we can access information from your nervous system in real time, we can use lab results to guide our testing. It's like the lab test is a high-resolution map under the "GPS" of our nervous system testing.

What we find out by testing:

- What area your body wants to heal next (We call this the *priority*).
- What other areas of your body are stressed, and to what degree.
- What is causing the stress.

With this information, we can work with your body to help it make progress in healing.

What do labs show?

- In most cases, a lab won't show the reason for the test result. For example, your cholesterol could show as high, but the lab can't say *why* this is. The *why* is what nervous system testing tells us.

- Lab values are usually *relative*. This means that the value itself may be good or bad, but the meaning of the lab depends on other information, such as other lab values, health history, symptoms, etc.
- All labs are snapshots. The lab can only show the information available in the moment it was done. This information can be very valuable as a snapshot, but in most cases, follow-up labs are needed to get the full information. It's the difference between a picture and a video.

How are labs used?

Labs give us objective measures in very specific areas of your body to help us with:

- Determining when a patient should change the acupressure program they are doing and when it's OK to stop acupressure therapies and move to a supplement-only or booster program.
- Determining specific supplements a patient should be taking, and when they can stop taking other supplements.
- Showing stability of healing in a patient, allowing us to make an accurate decision on moving the person off active treatment to a wellness program.

We use labs in many ways.

Labs are critical in making decisions on the correct patient treatment program.

Example: A patient is just finishing their first three months (a cellular healing cycle) on a program. This patient had come to us complaining of fatigue, sleep problems, digestive problems, allergies, menstrual difficulties, and severe headaches. At their twelve-week reevaluation, the patient reported that many of their symptoms were much better, but several had persisted or still happened occasionally. Now, we must decide:

- Do an allergy program?
- Do a digestive protocol?
- Do a female hormone protocol?
- Do an adrenal protocol?

Only one choice is correct and will result in rapid healing and a happy, recovering patient. *How do we decide? We must either use labs to help us . . . or guess.*

Labs are also important in making correct decisions about which supplements to recommend. We can test the nervous system to find which supplements the body can use and which it can't, but the possible combinations and priorities along with the limits on the number of supplements any patient can tolerate at once means that *we must either use labs to help us... or guess.*

To get good results, we must support the body. *Bodies are dynamic and alive and changing all the time. We must see and measure what's changing so we can know what to do next.*

Follow-up labs save you money.

The way to save money on any treatment program is to *make it shorter.* We have patients who have refused to do follow-up labs for the past ten years and who are still buying supplements and paying for visits. With these patients, all we can do is to try to keep their symptoms under the best control possible. Without the information from labs, that's all we can do. *The patient will never recover enough to move off an active program, or even to reduce supplements. We're just "holding the fort" forever.*

Doing follow-up labs as soon as possible after we recommend them to you will save you money and health.

Study Question Box 6

1. Think of a time when you failed to predict a problem and had a very stressful experience because of this (didn't save for a rainy day, etc.). You can share if you like!

2. *Overheard at a tire store:* Customer: "I'm sure my bald tires are fine for another 100,000 miles at least. What benefit would I get if I bought new tires?" Salesman: "Your car will ride and handle somewhat better." Customer: "I can't see spending $600 just so my car handles a little better." *What should the salesman say to the customer to save his life if the customer cannot be convinced that his bald tires will cause him a problem?*

The Truth

What is really required to regain and maintain your health once you've had a significant chronic health condition?

Chronic health problems come from your body not being able to heal itself, and the only solution lies in actions that *you* take to reduce stress and assist healing until your body recovers its healing ability . . . and then heals itself.

You have been living in your body all your life and *so are responsible for the condition that it's in right now.*

"Responsibility" means "cause." If you cause something, you are responsible for what you caused.

- If you have caused something, there is an excellent chance that you can do something effective to reverse the situation and remedy any bad effect from it.
- On the other hand, if you think you are a victim and have no responsibility for your condition, then you might have a lot of difficulty changing it.

Our experience has always been that if a patient takes responsibility for their health, and they are willing to do whatever is necessary to resolve "their own" health problems, they get well!

Those patients who don't feel they are responsible for their health are often easily convinced that they are "all better" when they've just started healing. They may crave a "fix-me" type solution and want to find a treatment or supplement that will resolve their problems without having to alter their lifestyle or spend time or finance. In a way, it's kind of a get-rich-quick mentality.

To Sum It Up

The cheapest, fastest solution to a chronic health problem is to handle the hell out of it with the highest priority for effort, time, and money— until the problem is gone and **labs indicate that your health is fully stable**. Then you should continue to live a lifestyle that supports whatever level of stress control is needed to keep your body stable for the rest of your life.

If this just isn't possible, then second-best is that you live a lifestyle that won't stress your body (diet, activity, sleep, avoid toxic people, etc.), and do a basic program with us to gradually improve your health instead of having it slip backwards.

If you don't do either, my experience is that you may well fight various and worsening chronic conditions for the rest of your life. The expense can be astronomical. The damage to your quality of life, relationships, and productivity can't be measured.

There I go again, sounding all dire. I wish it wasn't so true.

Study Question Box 7

1. Name some actions or inactions you have taken during your life that have contributed to your current health problems.

2. Name three benefits to addressing a health condition earlier rather than later when it becomes much worse:

   1.

   2.

   3.

3. Name three examples of things that will get better or worse but will not stay the same for long:

   1.

   2.

   3.

The Secret to Good Health

Isn't this what everyone is looking for? I don't want to leave you hanging without handing this over to you as a gift.

This secret is just one observation: *everything in the universe gets better or worse— nothing stays the same for long.*

This applies to health. If you continue to take effective actions to cause your health to improve, your health will continue to get better. If you decide that your "health is good" and you go back to "life as normal," thinking that your health will just continue . . . it won't.

When I talk about "stable health," what I mean is health that has improved to the point that it's possible for the patient to successfully work to keep it improving continually without any extraordinary help from us.

A person with "stable health" can continue to improve that health (and thus stay healthy) with the following actions, *done for the rest of their lives*:

Actions Necessary to Continue to Improve Your Health

1. Eat in a way that does not stress your body.

2. Take the correct (tested) dietary supplements needed to support weak areas of your body and prevent deterioration.

3. Have an active lifestyle that involves significant motion several times a day (doesn't have to be "exercise," can just be walking for 30–45 minutes a day).

4. Avoid severe lifestyle stresses: exposure to high levels of toxins, association with toxic personalities, insufficient sleep, etc.

5. Get tested at the correct intervals to catch any problems that are developing. This would be Evectics[SM] testing, functional lab tests, appropriate medical testing.

Does this seem like too much trouble to go to? If so, remember the "secret." *If you don't continually work to get better, you'll get worse.*

And continually better is what I want for you! I invite you to join the group of happier and healthier people who have avoided the medical traps and are living their lives with energy and vitality and without fear of serious health problems. Please take me up on the offer!

Study Question Box 8

From the list of actions needed to have stable health, check off the applicable boxes:

1. I eat in a way that does not stress my body.

   ❑ I do this now ❑ I will do this for the rest of my life ❑ I don't do this
   ❑ I'm doing this now but will likely stop.

2. I take the correct (tested) dietary supplements needed to support weak areas of the body and prevent deterioration.

   ❑ I do this now ❑ I will do this for the rest of my life ❑ I don't do this
   ❑ I'm doing this now but will likely stop.

3. I have an active lifestyle that involves significant motion several times a day (doesn't have to be "exercise," can just be walking for 30 – 45 minutes a day)

   ❑ I do this now ❑ I will do this for the rest of my life ❑ I don't do this
   ❑ I'm doing this now but will likely stop.

4. I avoid important lifestyle stresses: exposure to high levels of toxins, association with toxic personalities, insufficient sleep, etc.

   ❑ I do this now ❑ I will do this for the rest of my life ❑ I don't do this
   ❑ I'm doing this now but will likely stop.

5. I get tested at the correct intervals to catch any problems that are developing. This would be Evectics℠ testing as well as medical testing.

   ❑ I do this now ❑ I will do this for the rest of my life ❑ I don't do this
   ❑ I'm doing this now but will likely stop.

Study Question Box 9

Please write a short paragraph letting us know what you learned or gained from doing this course.

Do you have any suggestions of additions, deletions, or changes you think we should make in this course?

Thank You! *Congratulations on completing this book!*

www.ingramcontent.com/pod-product-compliance
Lightning Source LLC
Chambersburg PA
CBHW050346290526
45785CB00006B/2654